SMILING from EAR to EAR

WRITTEN & ILLUSTRATED BY

Kaitlyn Chu

For all of the courageous and selfless
heroes who are on the front lines

Special thanks to my Chu Crew
for being my lifeline

Smiling From Ear to Ear
Copyright © 2020 by Kaitlyn Chu

Published in the United States of America by Kaitlyn Chu.

ISBN 978-1-7352997-0-9

Website: www.lovechudesigns.com

Instagram: @lovechudesigns

Email: kaitlyn@lovechudesigns.com

Hey there!

Let's keep each other safe
while having fun and smiling
from ear to ear!

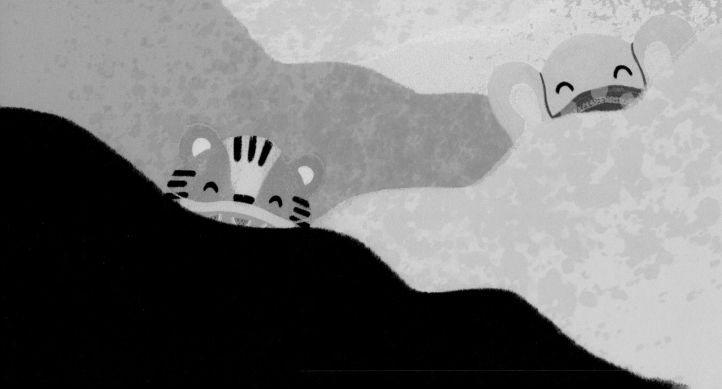

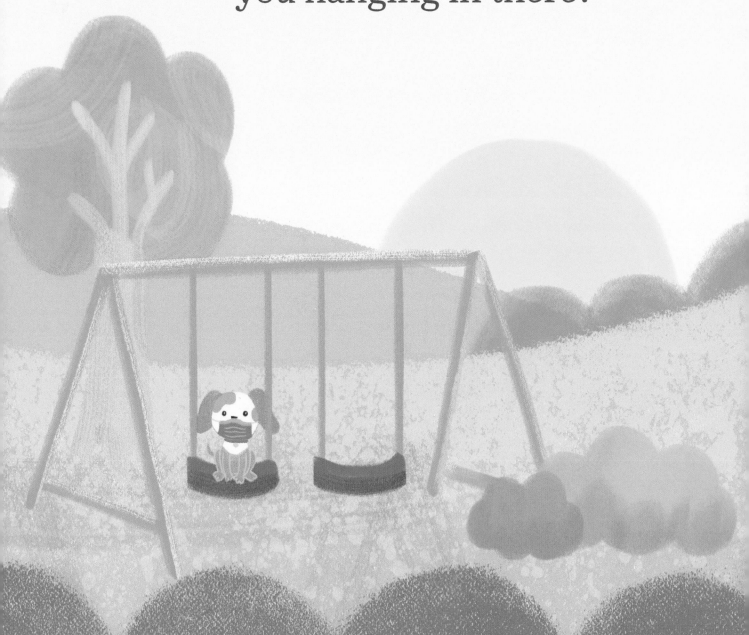

Hey playful monkey, how are you hanging in there?

I'm having fun even with
the mask I wear!

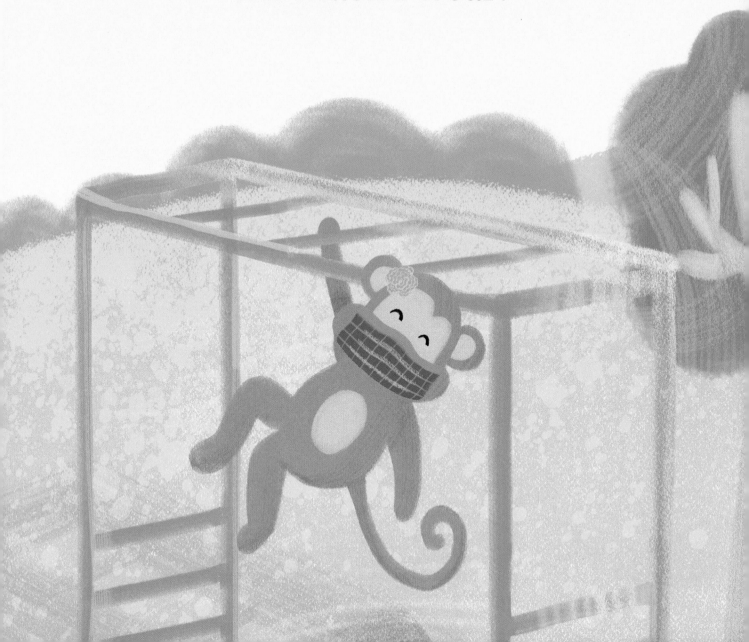

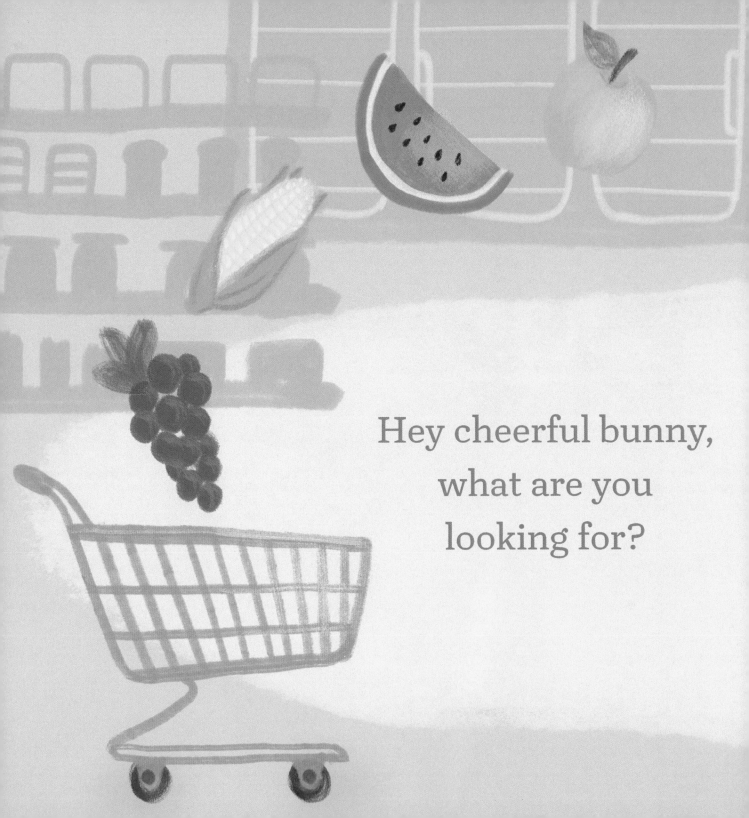

Hey cheerful bunny, what are you looking for?

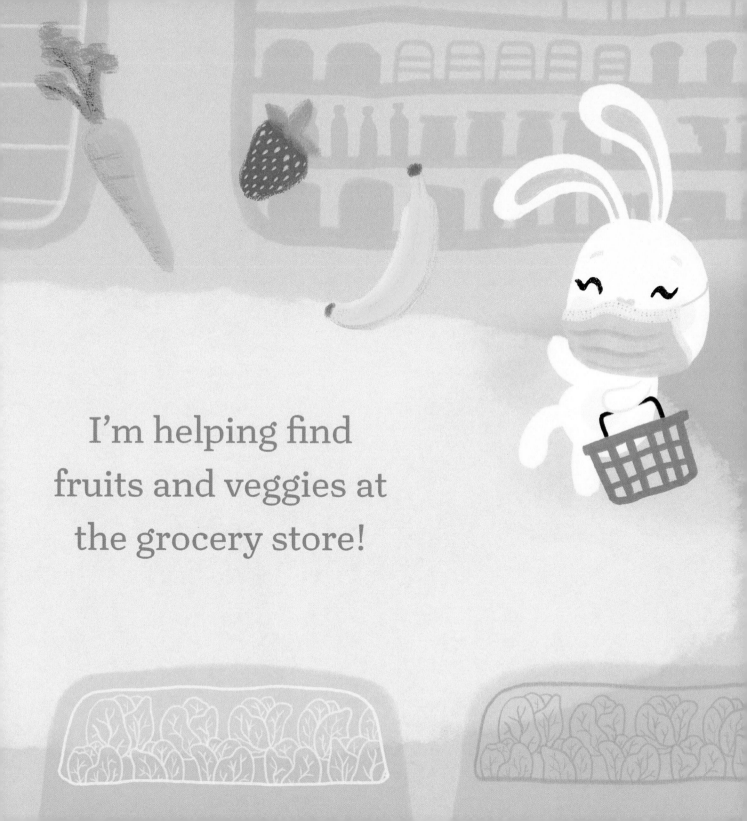

I'm helping find
fruits and veggies at
the grocery store!

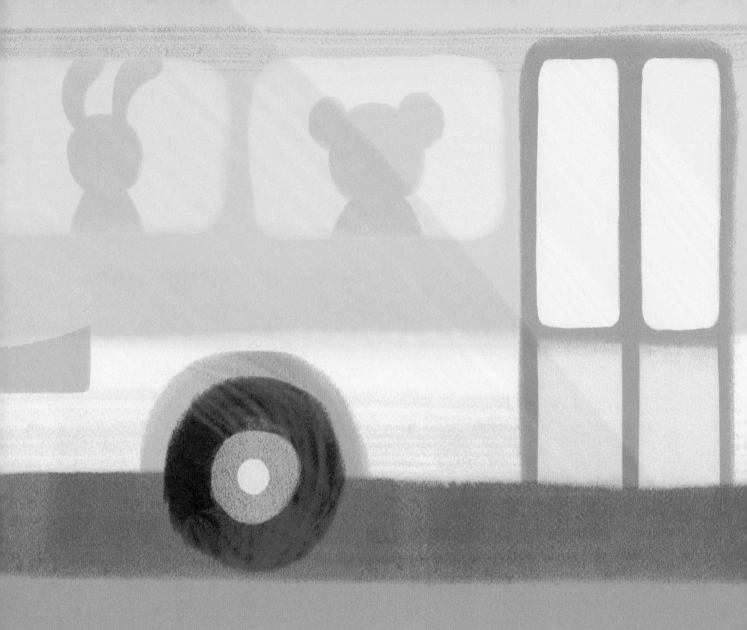

Hey sporty tiger, where
are you going on the bus?

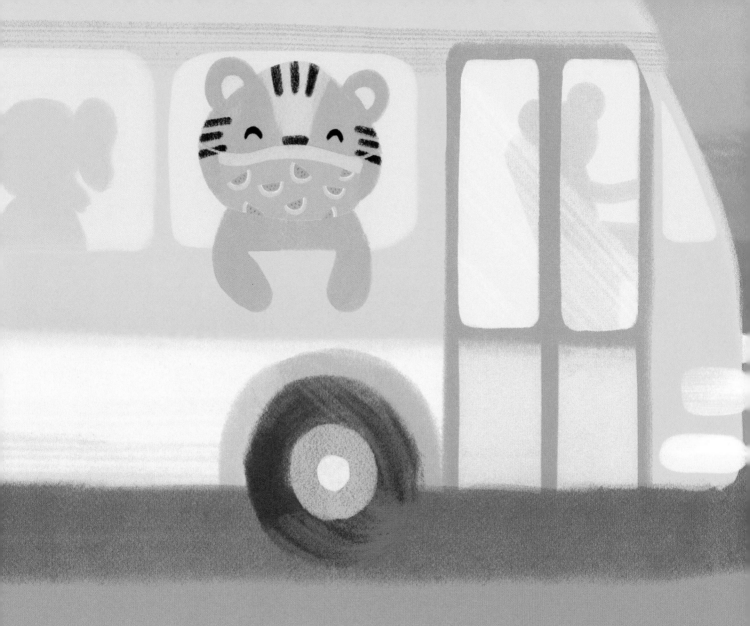

I'm heading to the park to
play ball — come join us!

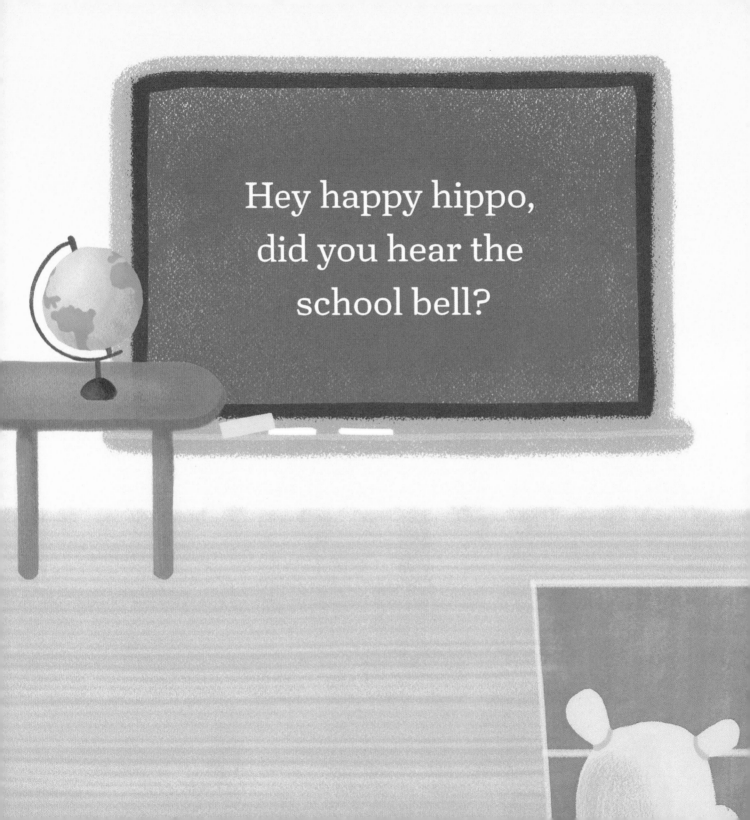

Hey happy hippo,
did you hear the
school bell?

Yes, and now it's time
for my show and tell!

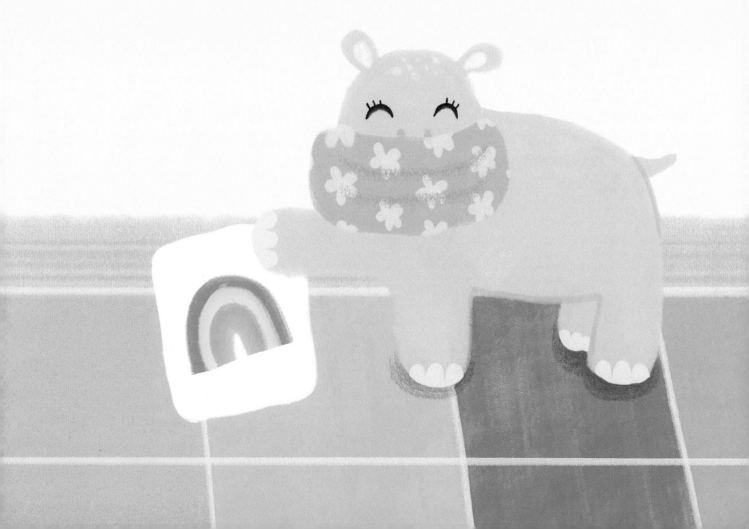

Hey sweet panda,
what are you
dreaming of?

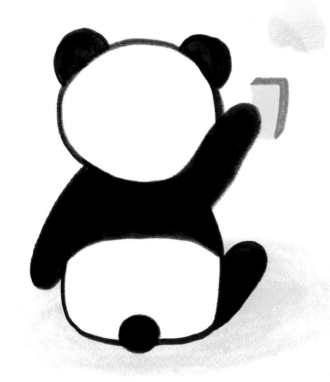

I'm finishing my
chores so I can go
eat a treat I love!

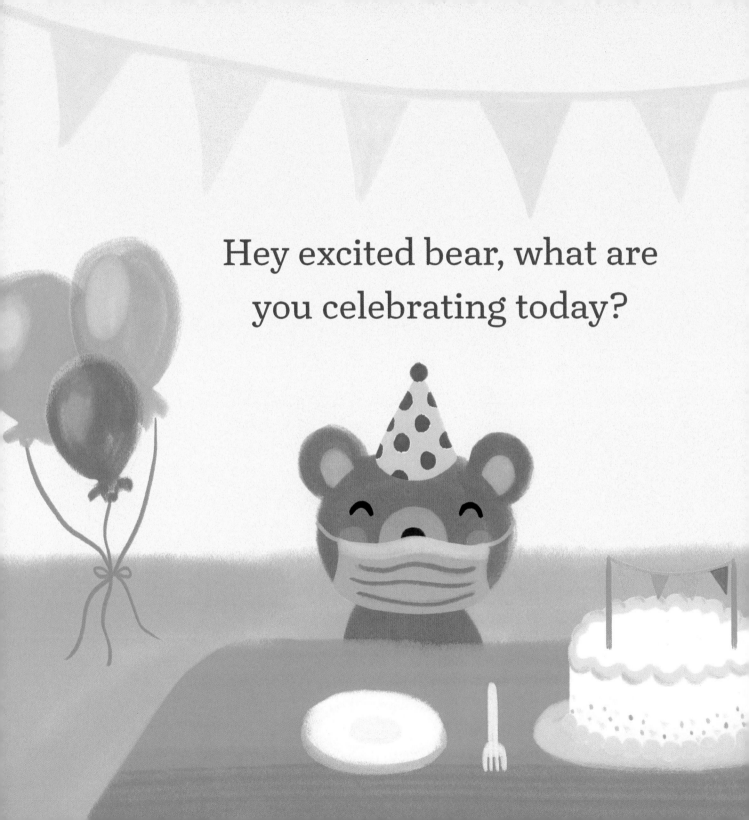

Hey excited bear, what are you celebrating today?

We are all here for my beary best friend's birthday!

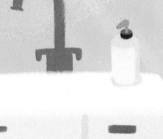
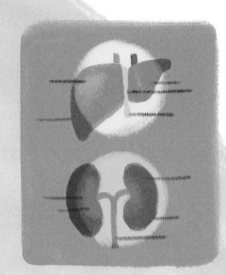
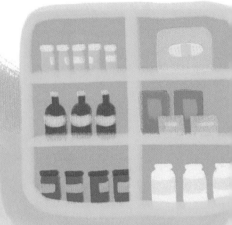
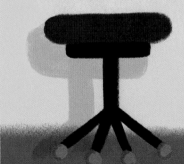

Hey courageous sheep,
who are you going to see?

I'm waiting for the
doctor to check up on me!

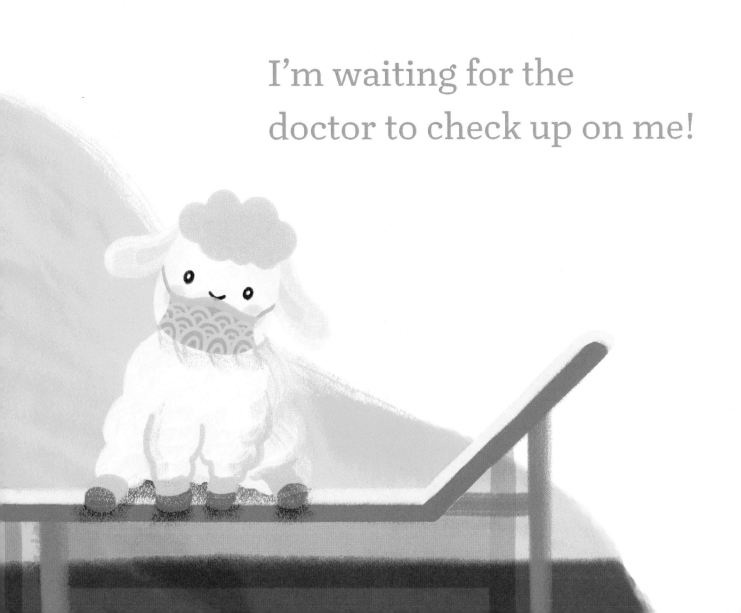

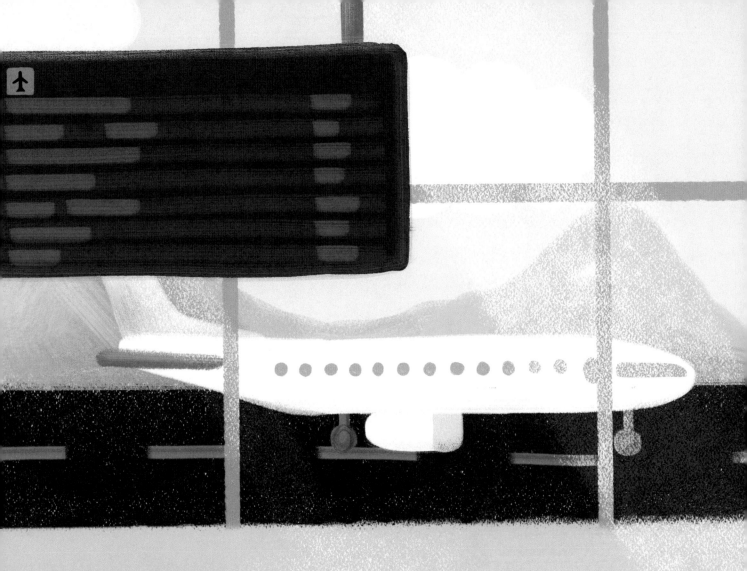

Hey adventurous frog,
are you ready to fly?

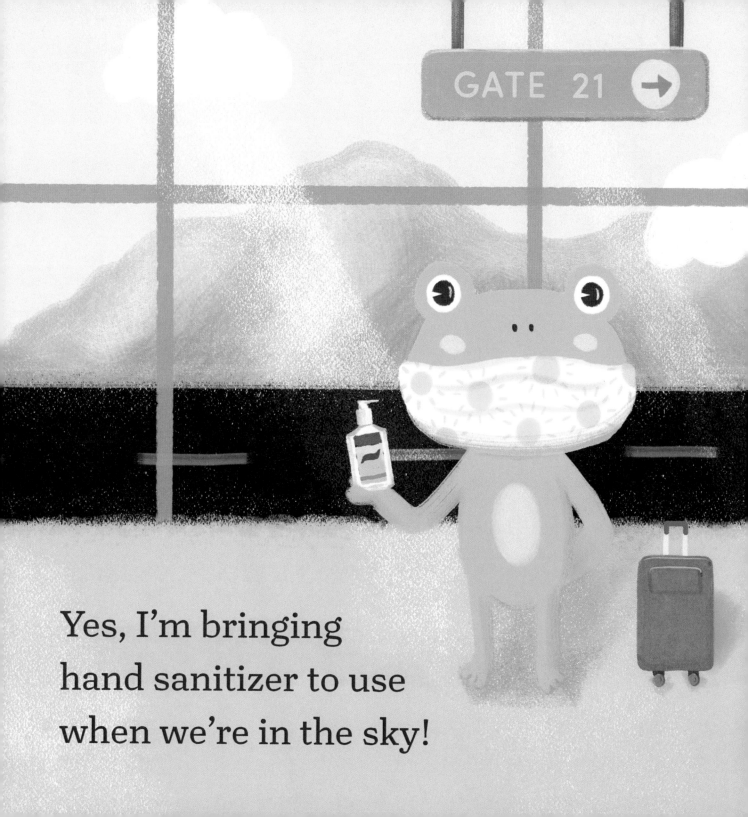

Yes, I'm bringing hand sanitizer to use when we're in the sky!

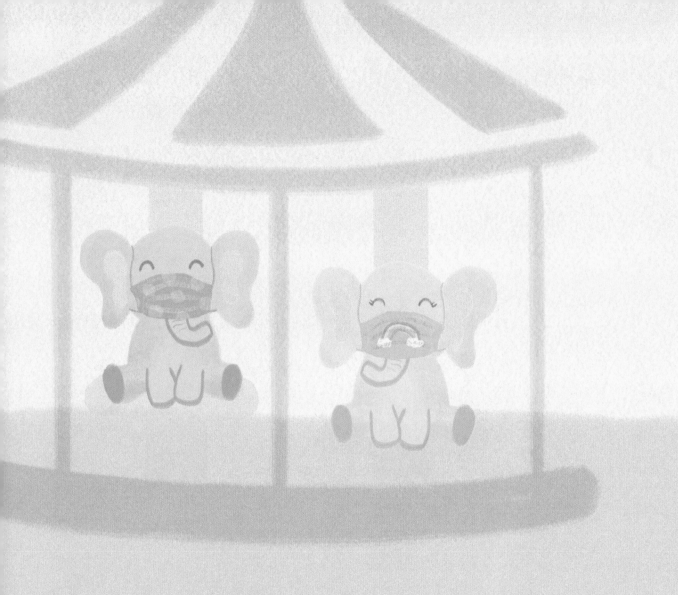

Hey fun-loving elephant,
what is your favorite ride?

I'm happiest when
I'm racing down
the giant slide!

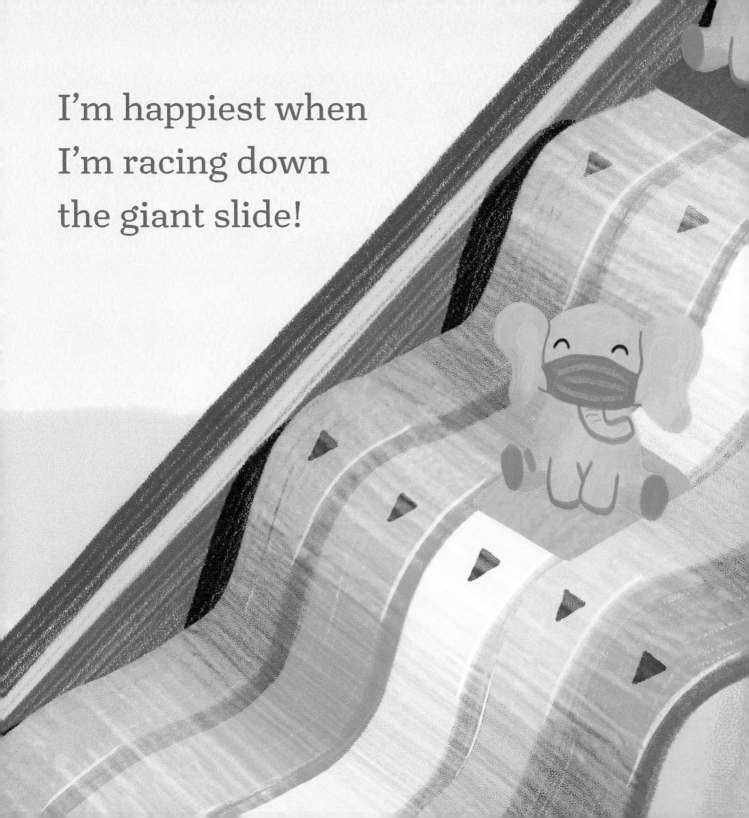

Hey caring giraffe,
who are you here to see?

I'm visiting my supportive
extended family!

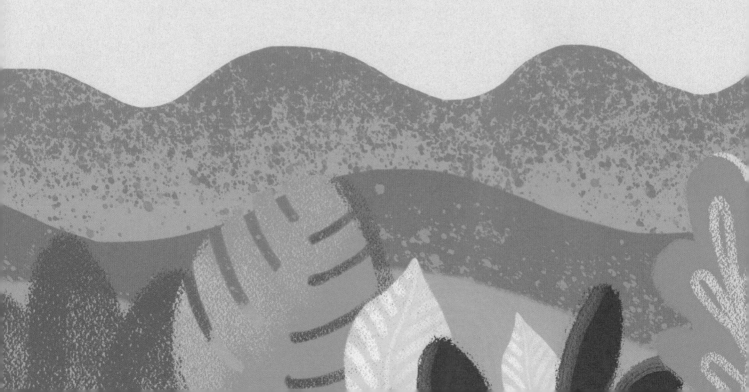

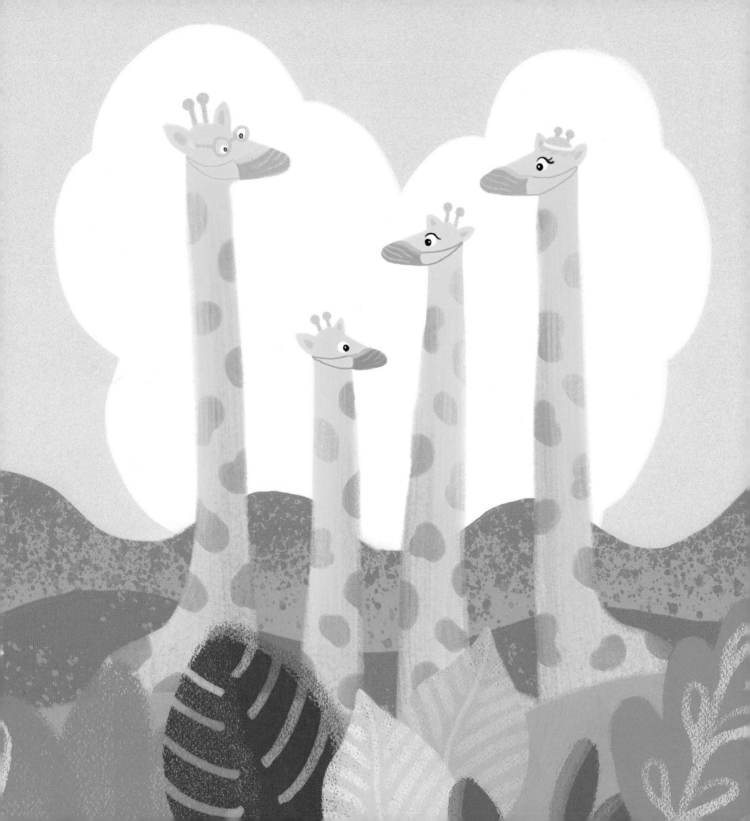

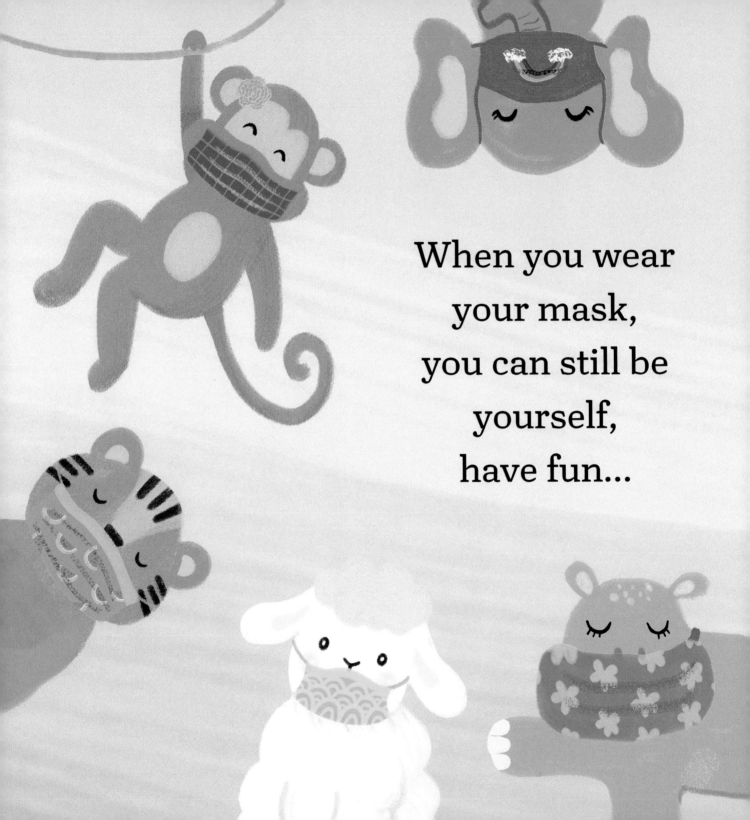

When you wear
your mask,
you can still be
yourself,
have fun...

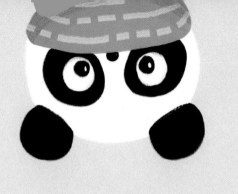

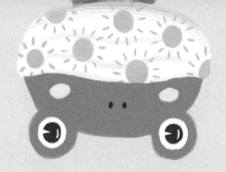

and most importantly,
protect yourself and your
loved ones! We're all smiling
from ear to ear. Let's see you
smile with your mask on!

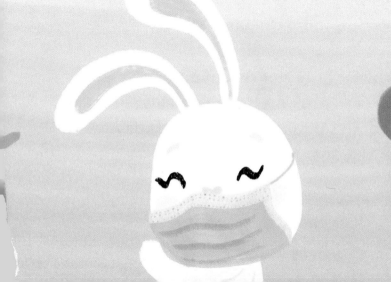

ABOUT THE AUTHOR | ILLUSTRATOR

Kaitlyn Chu

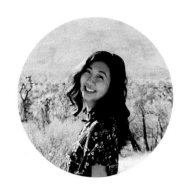

HEY THERE!

Thank you so much for supporting my book and its mission to show kids that they can wear face masks to protect themselves and those around them and still have fun. I wanted to address kids' fears and struggles by normalizing face masks in everyday activities using a playful and imaginative approach.

I'm from Orange County, CA and am a senior at the University of Southern California studying Arts, Technology and the Business of Innovation. I have always loved expressing myself creatively through designing: user experiences, consumer products and community programming. For fun I enjoy visiting Disneyland, spending time with friends & family, and playing escape room games.

My goal is to positively impact lives through everything I do in a fun, happy and accessible way. I do this by taking action on current issues through mediums including children's books, websites, videos, graphics and community organizations.

EMAIL: kaitlyn@lovechudesigns.com | IG: @lovechudesigns | lovechudesigns.com

Made in the USA
San Bernardino, CA
07 August 2020